Weight Loss

Balanced Eating for Fat Burning and Muscle Keeping

Table Of Contents

Introduction.

I want to start by thanking you for purchasing my book **"Weight Loss: Balanced Eating for Fat Burning and Muscle Keeping".**

It is common to see health advice in various media advocating the importance of eating healthy and becoming more physical active. This is actually easy to say, but it is very important to be proactive when it concerns matters of health and fitness.

It is good to promote the need for physical activities to be included in our daily routine, it is necessary for good health and also to fight against becoming obese or suffering many other health challenges. As much as we should engage in physical activities, we should also recognize the fact that we need to support our healthy lifestyle with the right eating habit. It will become quite retrogressive if we dedicate ourselves to becoming physically active while we still eat unhealthy foods.

The best way to lose weight is to moderate the quantity and the quality of food you eat together with having a good exercise routine. You also need to eat moderately and become physically active to control your weight.

It is possible to eat as much as you want and still maintain a healthy lifestyle while looking fit and trim. This contrasts the proposed notions that you must reduce your food intake for foods high in carbohydrates before you can lose weight.

It is easy to get confused with the numerous diets and health advice you will get from the media and other sources. I should stress here that cutting a particular food from your diet is not the answer. What you need to do is create a diet that includes only healthy foods that will ensure you are in good health without unnecessary weight gain.

We need to clearly define what a balanced diet is. A balanced diet is one that contains the necessary nutrients your body needs to function properly in their right proportions. A balanced diet will contain all the forms of nutrients. Nutrients can be grouped into micro and macro nutrients. Micronutrients include vitamins and minerals, while macronutrients include protein, carbohydrates, and the fats. They all complement each other to provide the human body with the enough nourishment and energy, this is essential for a healthy life.

It is possible to lose weight by reducing the number of carbohydrates and calories consumed. Your body will find fewer bad fats and sugars to process; this will aid a better metabolism. Many healthy diets are created in line with increasing the vegetable content while attempting to completely remove processed foods and foods rich in simple carbohydrates from the menu. It will be a good thing if this works for many people who might be used to the unhealthy western diets we have now.

Step 1. Know your enemy!

Western diets are usually packed with so unhealthy fats, and simple carbohydrates that constitute a very heavy diet; this gives the digestive system challenges to process the consumed food. In the long run, eating like this will make you look older and less attractive; these kinds of meals should be avoided.

The groups of foods that we should avoid have been tagged badly because they either contain toxic compounds or they are packed full with sugars and Trans fats.

Saturated fats are not very good, what are worse are the Trans fats. Trans fats are unhealthy and extremely harmful to our bodies. Policies are underway to completely eliminate the use of Trans fats in our food industry.

What makes Trans fats so bad? Trans fats are oils that have hydrogen molecules in their structure. They are responsible for promoting the production of bad cholesterol and they also influence the actions of cells working in the body from performing their normal functions. Trans fats distort the hormonal balance in the human body, this can set off abnormalities and other ailments like cancer, stroke, and infertility etc. the source of Trans fats include fried foods, baked foods, and processed food.

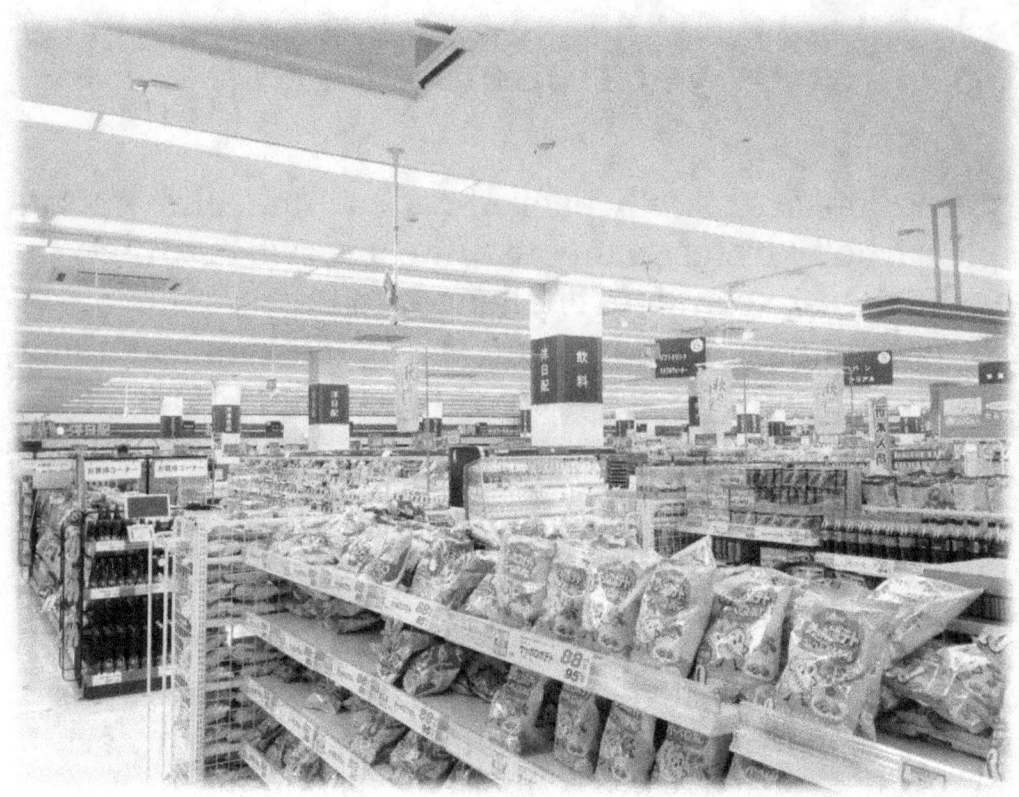

Processed Foods. These are those brightly packaged foods that you see on the shelves in shops, they are mostly canned foods, packaged meats, frozen meals. Processed foods contain everything we need to avoid. They are mostly packed with salt and high in calories. The labels are created to be somewhat deceptive as you can see written on the label "low fat" these foods are actually packed with harmful trans-fat. Just one serving can contain the total amount of sodium or calories that you are required to take the entire day, and most times one serving is never enough to satisfy you. Unfortunately, they are the cheapest foods in the market. This can be very enticing, but you should consider the long term effects like cancer and other ailments. This should be enough scare to keep you away from buying them.

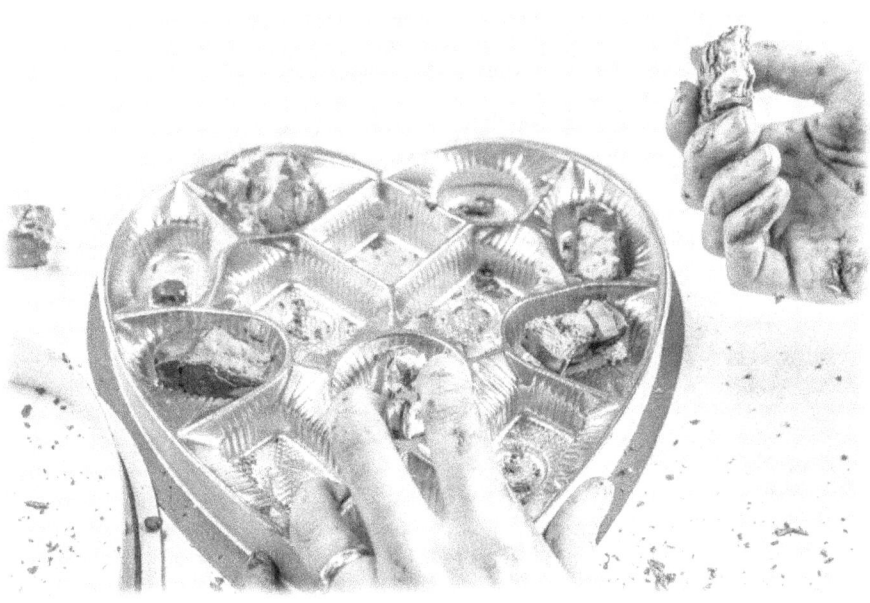

Candies and sweetnesses. These foods have been proven to have a remarkably positive effect on your mood. Caution should be used when including candies and sugar treats in your meals because they are packed with high amounts of sugar. It is a good thing that candies are usually packaged in small wraps, but they can still be abused especially by people with large appetites.

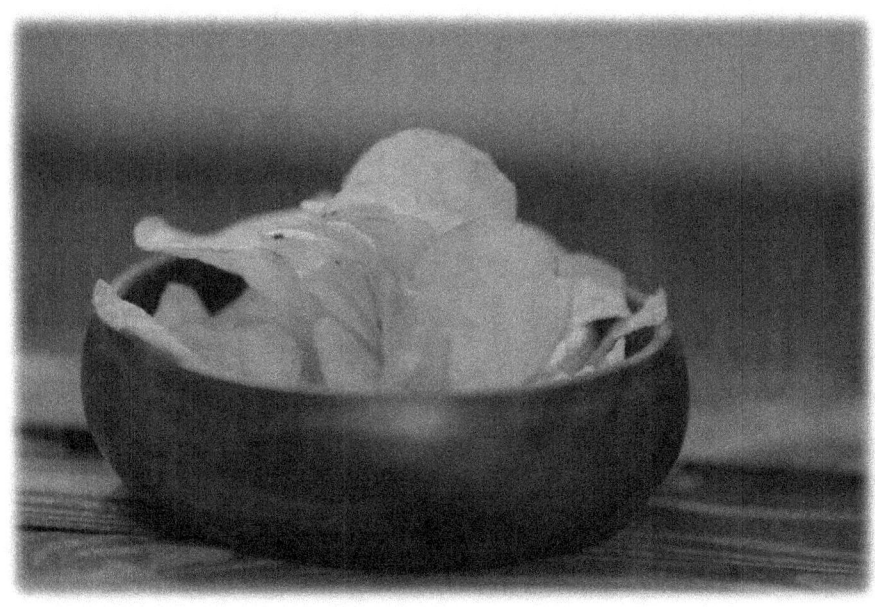

Potato chips are known to contain harmful Trans fats and hydrogenated oils. They are also packed with salt. Please avoid these foods. Fortunately, there are many other options of snacks to choose from if you are feeling slightly hungry.

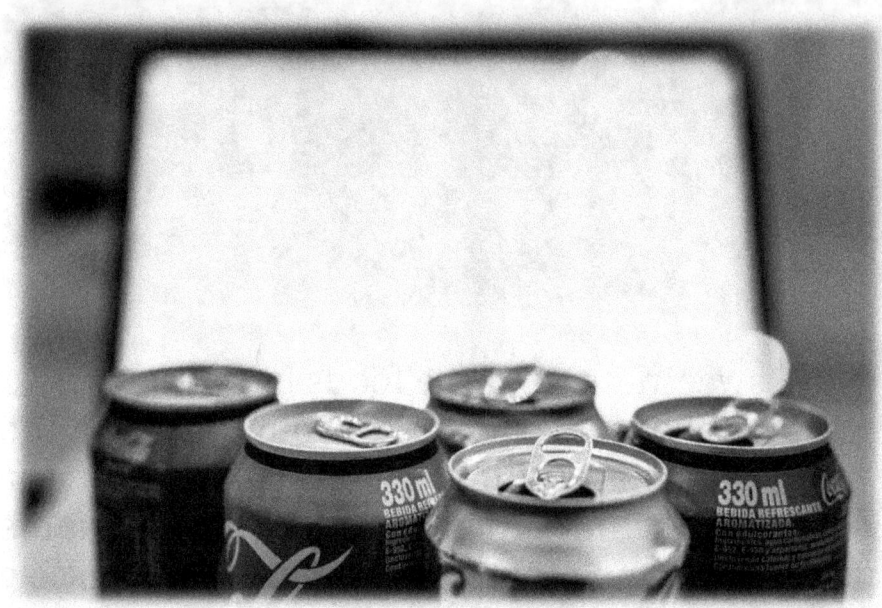

I know this might be given the "side eye" but sodas are not healthy drinks. They contain huge amounts of sugar and this can shoot your blood sugar levels to alarming heights. Some sodas have been tagged as "diet soda". There might have been a reduction in the sugar content, but we can never know how much, a soda drink is always packed with sugar. Why not choose to drink water especially if you are trying to lose weight.

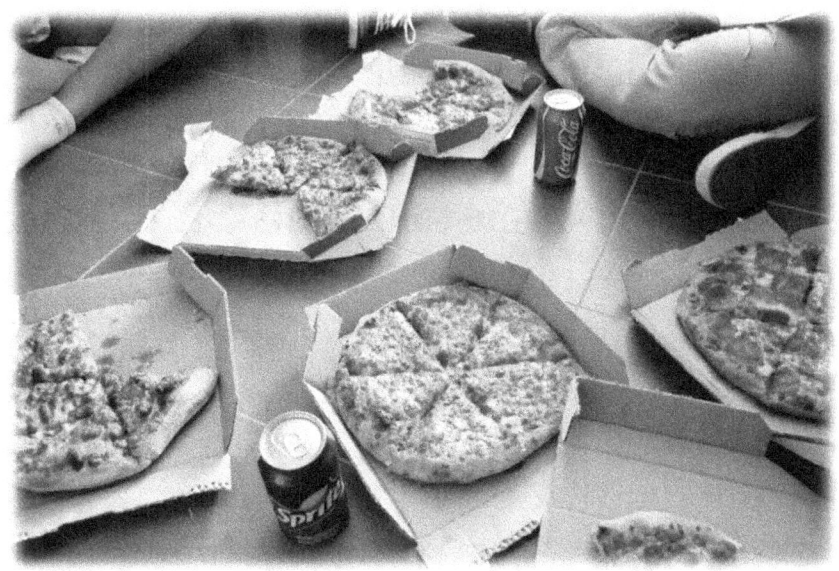

Fast foods are one of the biggest challenges to planning a healthy eating habit. They include burgers, pizza, and some Chinese foods. Fast foods are packed with trans-fat and they have very high-calorie content. You should strive to find other foods that will substitute fast foods in your menu if you are one of those people who have regular seats in a fast food restaurant. It is good that healthy fast food restaurants have started springing up everywhere. This will make it easier for those fast food lovers.

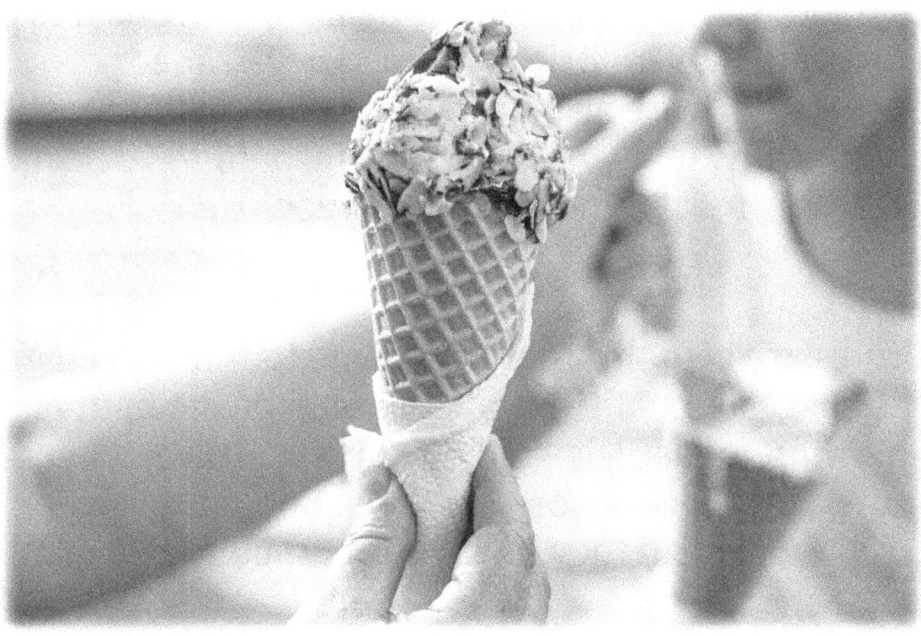

Yes, ice cream and milkshakes are sweet, too sweet and very tempting. They will make you add more weight than you ever imagined in a very short while. They are also packed with unsaturated fats. Just one serving can contain as much as 1,000 calories so you should consider taking these foods in moderation.

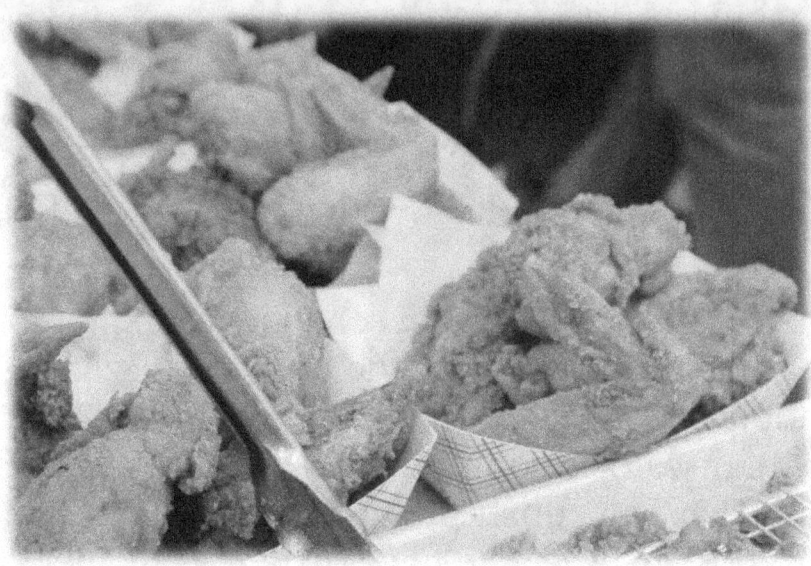

Fried foods basically refer to foods that have been prepared by frying in oil and packaged for sale to the end consumers. They include donuts, fried chicken, onion rings, French fries, etc. fried foods are packed with the harmful Trans fats and they have very high-calorie content. The dreaded hydrogenated oils are also part of the contents of most fried foods. Ironically, many of these foods would have been part of a nutritious meal if they have not been fried.

Substitutes are actually an ironic name that has been given to foods suggested to the public that can be eaten in place of other harmful foods. They include artificial sweeteners, salt substitutes, artificial flavors, and oils. Substitutes are processed foods, and they have the characteristics of all processed foods. You will be doing your body a very good service to avoid these substitutes.

Low-Fat Foods. It is a good thing that the manufacturers of "low fat" foods are being at least truthful. From the name tag, it is obvious that there is fat in the foods and we hate fats. Unfortunately, many foods termed as low fat contain huge amounts of other foods that are not healthy. Low-fat foods include cookies, salad dressings, yogurt etc. please be on the safer side and choose organic foods to processed "low fat foods".

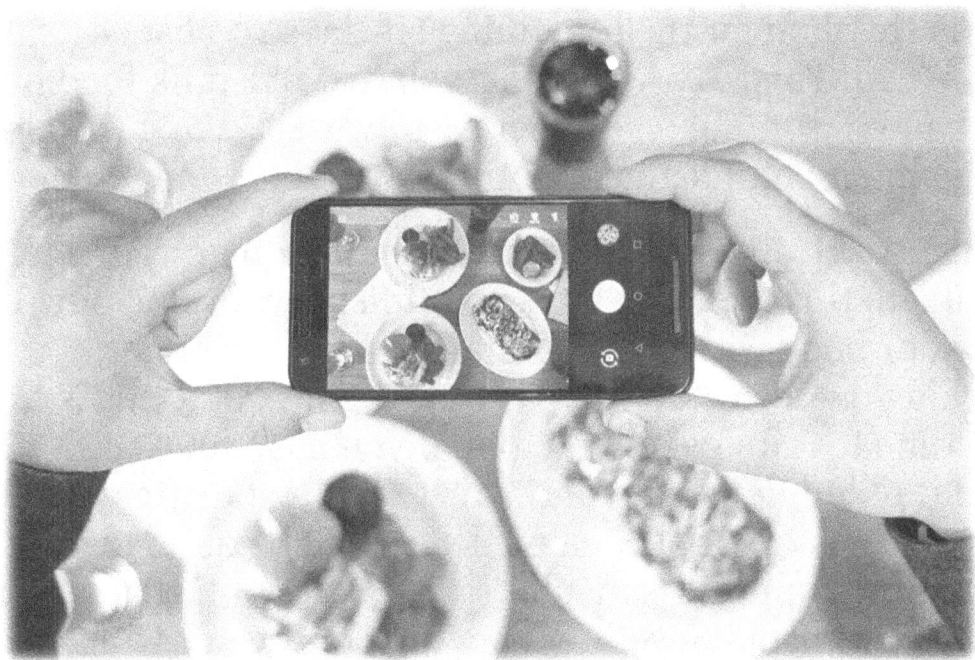

The foods served in restaurants are notorious for containing alarming amounts of calories. Restaurants offer a large menu to their customers. Many people love to dine in restaurants and usually pick their foods from a menu that has not broken down the actual contents in terms of calorie content and the methods of preparation. There is good news; many restaurants have adopted healthy menus as many people are becoming increasingly aware of the harmful effects of unhealthy eating habits.

I know a lot of you might be very troubled at the moment because many of these foods that have been labeled as harmful have become a major part of your daily feeding habit. You do not have to worry; there is something that can easily be done about his.

I have a plan that will make you very happy and you will not have to feel the burden of guilt that you are cheating. What if you indulge yourself for just one day out of the seven days in a week? Does this sound good? You can set aside a day to eat all the foods that you crave, ice cream, donuts, burgers, and pizzas etc. then for the remaining six days you eat as healthy as you can. This way, you will still have your junk food but you will be working on a progress towards leaving the old eating habit behind and adopting a better and healthier diet.

I will also let you know the best time to indulge yourself. You should do this after you have just finished working out. This way your body will be able to handle the food better. Working out also stabilizes your hormones, and this is the best time to indulge in junk food if you have to. Another benefit of indulging in your favorite junk food after working out is because your adrenaline levels will be quite high, adrenaline suppresses insulin so you will not have to bother about your insulin levels spiking up. However, I will advise you to avoid processed foods and foods contain high Trans fats if you have to indulge in sweets and unhealthy foods. Whatever you eat will be quickly absorbed into your system without depositing those bad fats.

Step 2. Drink water!

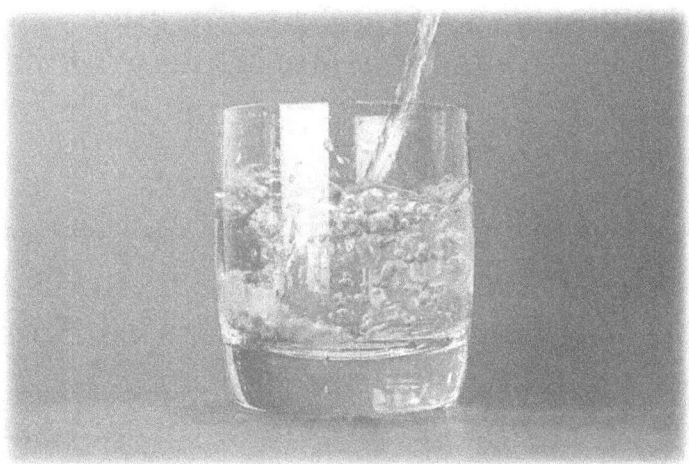

Water makes up about 50% of our bodies. We all need water to survive; this is obvious because just feeling a little bit dehydrated with cause you to have a little headache if you continuously deprive yourself of water. You need to constantly drink water to replace lost fluids.

The following are some interesting facts about water:

Dehydration (lack of water) is the primary reason for fatigue.

Dehydration reduces your metabolism.

Water can be used to get relief from hunger temporarily.

Statistics have shown that Americans do not drink enough water; they mostly misconstrue thirst for hunger and end up eating their meals with sodas.

Studies have shown that drinking as much as 8 glasses of water daily will provide relief for joint aches.

Drinking water will balance out the effects of alcohol and other beverages. It will also replenish fluids lost from the body after exercise or from sweating.

Keep drinking water until your urine is clear or light yellow.

A good advice for those of you that work out is to avoid drinking too much water before your workout sessions. You should drink plenty of water before and after your workout sessions. Drinking too much water while working out can cause cramps to set in, your system can also become irritated.

Do you know that water can also help you lose weight? This is how it works, the liver breaks down fats in the body and it functions better when you are well hydrated. So drinking enough water will help your liver to work at its best capacity thus breaking down and getting rid of unwanted fat.

Water can be consumed at any time of the day when you feel like you have not had enough already. There is no substitute for water. Your body will react in an unpleasant and irritable way if you deprive it of water. Drinking water in the morning boosts your body's metabolism. The recommended pattern for drinking water is a glass every hour. You should adhere to this as much as you can.

Your meals should contain all the necessary nutrients.

This means that every meal you have should have the foods that will provide the necessary nutrients in the right quantity. It is important for you to know the daily recommended amounts of the basic nutrients.

A number of macronutrients should be higher, they are-

- Protein (good for muscle growth, repair and development)

- Carbohydrates (important for energy).

- Fats (good source of energy and supports organ functions)

The micronutrients are needed in smaller quantities, they include-

- Vitamins & minerals (vital for boosting the immune system and proper organ functions, cell development)

- Fiber (aids digestions)

The easiest way to ensure that your body is getting the right amount of nutrients and all the nutrients you need is to eat a wide variety of foods regularly.

Step 3. Grab your guidelines for protein consumption!

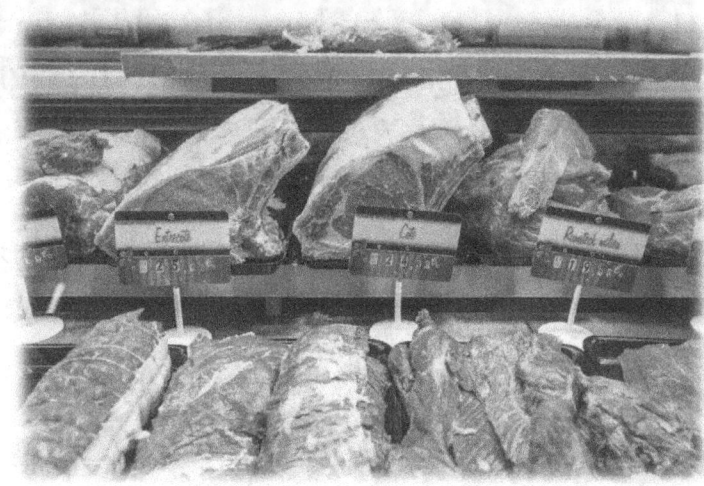

Protein is an important nutrient that helps to body to repair worn out tissues and muscles. Protein also facilitates muscle development and growth in every part of the body. We need some amounts of protein daily because our bodies do not store protein. A high amount of protein can lead to dehydration so it's best to plan your diet accordingly with the protein supplying foods.

Our bodies will get the best benefits from protein if we take it in the right amounts and in its most naturally occurring state.

Sources of protein include animals and plants. Protein is best in its most natural form; this means we should avoid processed protein foods as much as we can.

The recommended meat for a good source of protein is lean meat. Lean meat has little fat attached to it. It can be bought in the market or prepared by removing the fats from it. Cooking methods like baking, broiling, grilling and roasting are excellent for lean meat.

We have all been schooled about the dangers of red meat, but the reports have not been actually correct about red meat. It is as good as white meat. If you choose to eat lean red meat, you will not suffer the consequences attached to the red meat. It has been linked to many kinds of health challenges like cancer, stroke, and high blood pressure. Red meat is actually more nutritious than white meat, so you should go for lean red meat for a healthier diet.

I know many people will find this information relieving; you can enjoy your favorite red meat and still remain healthy. Other foods like seafood are classified as lean meat foods as well. The scare of high mercury content in seafood has created the need for caution. Mercury is dangerous to the brain and the nervous system. Always check with your seafood vendors to ensure that what they are selling is safe for consumption as you and your family will be at risk if it isn't.

Protein intake should be carefully planned to avoid taking too much protein. As we said earlier, protein is not stored in the body; it is also very slowly digested by our system. This means that you can check the amount of protein your diet contains. If you find yourself very hungry a couple hours after a meal, that meal had very little protein content. If you can stay without feeling hungry for up to 6 hours after a meal, then you should also check your protein content in your diet because it is too high.

Step 4. Reboot your metabolism with good carbs!

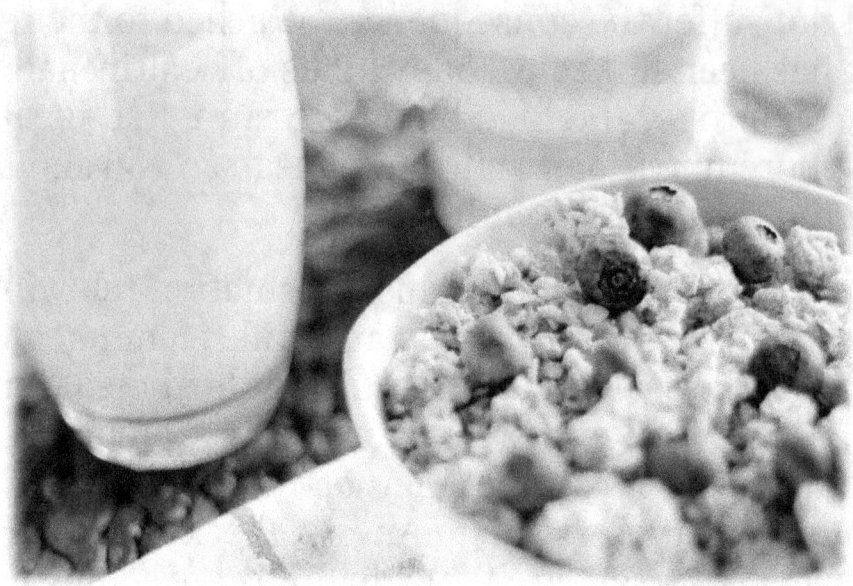

Carbohydrates provide your body with its most preferred form of energy. Carbohydrates are the major source of energy in our diet. It is essential that we get carbohydrates from our food but if it is present in very large quantities, it will lead to unwanted weight gain.

Carbohydrates are found in every other food that is not a source of proteins or fats. The major sources of carbohydrates include grains, cereals, fruits, pasta; bread etc., the main point to note here about this food nutrient is that only the good carbs should be included in your meals.

How do you make sure that your source of carbohydrate is the best for you?

Carbohydrates have an effect on your blood sugar levels. This is where you should start your investigation from. There are high and low glycemic carbohydrates. They have been classified like this due to the influence they have on blood sugar. High glycemic carbohydrates will have a little effect on the blood sugar level while low glycemic carbohydrates can spike up the blood sugar level to a dangerous point. The foods that contain this class of carbohydrates should be avoided.

Good carbs = complex carbs (low GI)

Bad carbs = simple carbs (high GI)

The simple carbohydrates are known as the high GI carbs. They are easily broken down by the body and they move into the blood stream to increase the sugar and insulin levels. This is usually what happens after a very large meal, the person suddenly feels drowsy and sleepy, and it is during the sleep that the excess sugar will be converted to fat in the body thereby causing an increase in weight.

A diet high in carbohydrates and sugar is not good for your health as you will be prone to heart diseases and diabetes. What you can do after a large meal is to remain as active as you can to help your body regulate the excess carbohydrates consumed.

On the other hand, the low GI carbohydrates are safer to consume. They are slowly broken down in the body; this is good because the amount of sugar introduced into the blood stream can be checked by this slow digestive process. The benefits are, a normal sugar level, generation of more energy by the body, and you can stay longer without feeling hungry.

Eating Low GI carbs (complex carbs):

The following benefits will be enjoyed when you eat low GI carbohydrates-

- It prevents you from feeling hunger soon after a meal.

- You will be able to manage your weight better.

- It improves blood cholesterol levels.

- Good stamina for sports.

Guidelines for consuming carbohydrates:

Your diet should be planned to exclude all forms of high glycemic carbohydrates. The sources of high glycemic carbs are sweets and processed carbohydrates. These foods have the characteristic sweetness that can make you long to eat them frequently. This makes it difficult to manage the consumption of high GI. A food item is defined as high GI if the total carbs content is more than the fat and protein content.

Never eat carbs alone. It is better to eat carbs with other foods that give proteins and/or healthy fats.

Your diet should be planned in a way that dinner has food items that contain low GI. This is because an abnormal increase in insulin will hamper the functions of the growth and repair hormones that are released while you are asleep.

If you cannot abstain from these carbs, you can fall back to setting a day aside just to indulge in your favorite sweets.

This means 6 days of the week will be dedicated to healthy eating and you can have fun on that appointed day. This is better in the long run because if you decide to have little quantities of carbs every day, in the long run, you stand the chances of relapsing back to the old ways of consuming a lot of unhealthy food unchecked.

The best combination of foods will be a mixture of high GI foods and proteins, feel free to include your favorite fats as well.

The high levels of adrenaline we have after exercising will create a window for consuming those carbs. The adrenaline will hamper the production of insulin, this means you can eat carbs and get away with it as it is absorbed into the body before the insulin levels become significant.

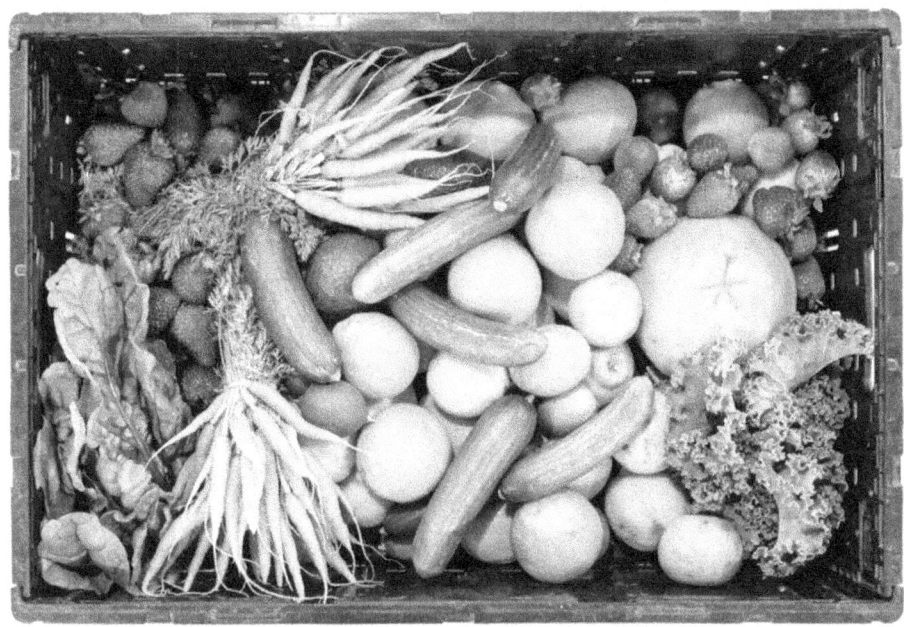

Our digestive system does not process fiber. This allows it to perform a cleansing function by carrying out all deposits from the digestive system through the intestines. Fiber foods make you feel full for longer periods after a meal. It also helps to check weight gain because it reduces the rate at which food is digested in the body. A good source of fiber is whole grains. Other sources are nuts, vegetables, fruits, wheat etc.

Step 5. Use Best Fats for Losing Fat!

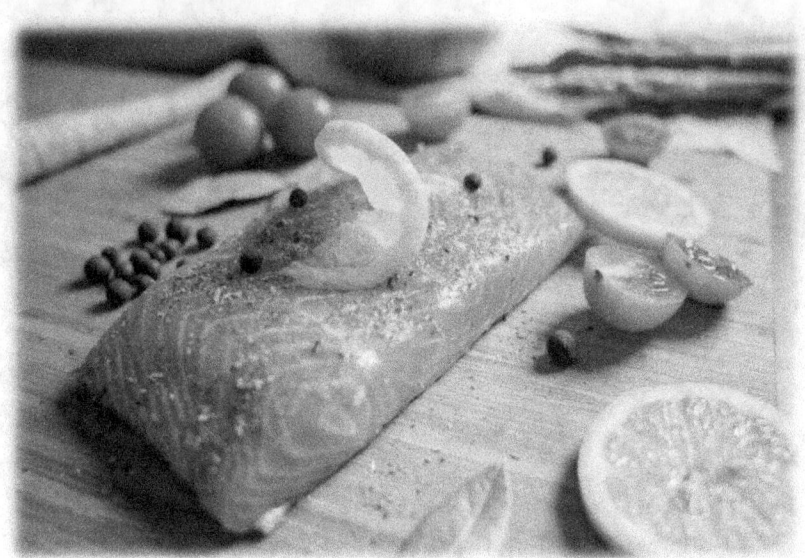

As much as we have identified fats to be the culprits behind unhealthy foods, our bodies need fats to function properly. Bad fats can cause health complications if they find their way into the arteries and clog them up. These kinds of fats can be avoided; you can eat fats and remain healthy with no harmful medical side effects.

The difference between good and bad fats:

• Good fats are classified as polyunsaturated and monosaturated fats. The sources of good fats include olive oil, cashews, almonds, nuts, seeds, fish, etc.

• Bad fats are classified as saturated fats, the sources of bad fat are predominantly from animal food products.

• Trans fats are the worst kind of fats. They are usually found in processed foods, fast foods, fried foods etc.

A god way to avoid eating too much is to include good fats in your meals. Fats make you feel full very quickly. Many people might be making the mistake of avoiding fats and thereby eating other foods which are also packed with harmful sugars and other unhealthy foods. You should include good fats in your meals; you will be able to check your eating habits to avoid overeating.

It is a good thing that the sources of good fats are foods that many of us will like. They are already a big part of our menus, and there is also room for them to be included if they are not on the menu already.

Guidelines for consuming fats:

Good sources that should be consumed regularly:

Omega-3 Fatty Acids (fish, seeds, nuts)

Omega-9 Fatty Acids (olive oil, avocado, etc.)

There should be caution when consuming these fats

Saturated Fats (full-fat dairy, heavily marbled or untrimmed cuts of animal protein)

Avoid the class by all means necessary:

Trans Fats and Hydrogenated Oils (fried/baked foods, chips, palm oil, processed foods)

Step 6. Timing beats ...weight!

If you are trying to watch your weight, you will be successful if you eat at the right time. The right time to eat is when your body will be able to easily digest and process the food without giving any chance for food to be stored as fat. If you can get this perfect times right, you will notice that your weight will not be influenced by the food you eat.

How much energy does the body need daily?

Your intake of foods should be synchronized with the way your body demands energy. This will be a good way to check the conversion of excess energy produced into fats. What you can do is to eat your meals close to the periods when you will engage in more activity thereby using up the generated energy.

Bad diet plan of eating only 3 big meals a day.

It is quite retrogressive to starve your body because you are trying to lose weight. I know you might have experienced how difficult it is to check your food intake when you finally decide to eat after starving your body. You will end up eating too much. You should always eat at regular times to avoid leaving too much time between meals.

It can be summed up as, starving yourself will decrease your body's metabolism, while the consequence of this will be over eating and this will lead to weight gain. Good diet plan of 6 meals a day

•Smaller portion of food will keep you satisfied all through the day and you will have enough energy for your activities.

•Snacks prevent hunger pangs and can be used to stall till you get to your meals.

Your meals should be planned to furnish your body with the right amounts of energy it needs at every given time. We always advise that breakfast should be large, and all other meals should be in smaller portions. This way, you will be able to manage your calorie intake. You can also have large meals before your workout sessions for the energy your body will get; this will be used up during a workout.

A good way to reduce your food intake will be to eat as many as 6 small meals evenly spaced throughout your day. This will keep hunger away and you should try to ensure that your meals if added up should be equal to on very large meal.

Start eating before you get too hungry. Stop eating before you get too full.

It is important that you eat a good breakfast. This is the first source of energy for your body and you will need this energy to start your day on a strong note. Skipping breakfast has many disadvantages. You will end up starving your body, the reaction will be a reduction in your body's metabolism and more fat will end up being stored making you gain weight. Ironic isn't it?

If you have to eat large meals before you work out, then you should also understand that this is done to provide energy during a workout. These meals should also be made up of foods that can be easily digested.

You can also snack a little after a workout. This can be followed by eating a good recovery meal. This will allow your body to go into a phase where the nutrient levels are balanced out making you feel better.

Avoid the urge to eat large meals after working out. This might be challenging but if you plan ahead and make the light foods ready as soon as you finish working out, you can avoid dealing with this urge because you will not be hungry.

It is a great idea to include fruits in your workout diets. They are a good source of vitamins. Eating a wide variety of foods will give you various forms of vitamins needed by the body to go through the workout session.

I mentioned earlier that you can indulge in some junk food if you find it almost impossible to stay away from them; this should be done after working out. This way your body easily absorbs the foods. I should also state here that this might go on for a while but you should not feel bad about your "weakness". It happens to everybody who starts out on this journey. The good news is that with time you will be able to overcome these urge and stick with eating only healthy foods. You will find the courage to focus on living and eating healthy when you start seeing the positive results.

Example sizes of snack meals:

Handful of nuts & 1 fruit

Handful of leafy greens & 1 hard-boiled egg

Pear with 1 oz. string cheese

Nutrition bar or protein bar

1 cup of nonfat plain Greek yogurt & 1/2 cup of fruit

Celery sticks with 1-2 tbsp. peanut butter

Eat very light dinner. This will give your system less work to digest food at night. Eating less during dinner is a good way to ensure that your meal is completely digested before you go to bed.

If you have to satisfy your hunger at night, you can have a little quantity of protein shake. This will take off any hunger pangs and get you through the night until it is time for breakfast.

Step7. Control your portions size!

Trying to determine how much you need to eat will ultimately depend on your body type. Different people have different needs, it works the same way as some people need to sleep for only a few hours at night and they are okay while others will need to sleep for long hours to get the needed rest.

A good place to start will be identifying how much energy you spend during your entire day, this will give you an idea of how much food you need to eat that will sufficiently provide this amount of energy for your body.

The next line of action will be for you to make a list of your favorite healthy foods and then determine which foods you will prefer to eat more. You should add these foods to your menu, the trick is to ensure that your body gets the necessary energy and nutrients and the right amount of foods to supply this energy and nutrients is included in your meals.

Using a nutrient ratio is another good way of keeping track of your nutrient consumption. It is easy to create and manage. You will get a good idea of your nutritional stance at a glance.

This is what a nutrient ratio looks like:

45-60% carbs

20-35% protein

10-25% fats

The Palm METHOD

This is a creative method that has been used for measuring food portions for a while. You will be able to estimate your meals in a way that you will eat regular portions of food during your meals. This is a good way to check over eating and also to balance your nutrients intake.

I know some people have very large palms, so this method should be used wisely. So you can easily add a little more to your pre-workout meals by measuring a few handfuls more of food. You can also ensure that your dinner is always very light.

Step 8. learn more weight loss tips!

If you are trying to lose weight, read this carefully. Always try to ensure that your daily calorie intake is balanced at values between 500-800 calories daily. This will be achieved by eating less and planning your meals accordingly or by using up more energy.

We can conclude by going over some basic things you have to do to live and eat healthy.

Your meals shouldn't contain less than 1,500 calories daily. This is an estimated value of calories that an adult needs to function properly all through the day. Do not ignore the importance of drinking water during your meals, and there is no substitute for water. You will be able to eat less if you eat slowly and try to stop eating before you start feeling full.

Try as much as you can to include only foods contain low GI in your menu, this might make you laugh but it helps to eat very well before you go grocery shopping. I know a lot of you will immediately connect with this statement. You will be able to resist buying unhealthy foods this way. Eat lots of fruits and vegetables, the fiber content and vitamins is very good for you. You can practice cooking your meals at home. This way you will have great opportunities to try out new recipes for cooking delicious healthy meals.

If you do not have junk food lying around you will have fewer challenges to refrain from eating them. You should avoid buying junk food; get your entire family to start eating healthy too. Fruits and nuts make excellent snacks that can help you go through hunger pangs. You should observe your cravings; it might be a sign that your body needs a particular vitamin.

I will also drop this advice here; Caffeine can provide your body with energy but it should be used with moderation. It can make you become dehydrated very quickly. Try to drink more water and eat fruits as well.

It might seem like a very long journey ahead, but you should start by setting long and short term goals. Your short term goals will indicate progress; this will make you happy and give you the courage to forge ahead. Your long term goals will be even more celebrated. When you start to see the positive results, you will become more determined not to spoil the good work you have started.

Conclusion

Make your food choices properly!

You are doing it for yourself!

Every day is yours!

Always!

Try these simple 8 steps for at least 30 days, see the results, and your life will be never same again. I hope this book will become a life changer for you.

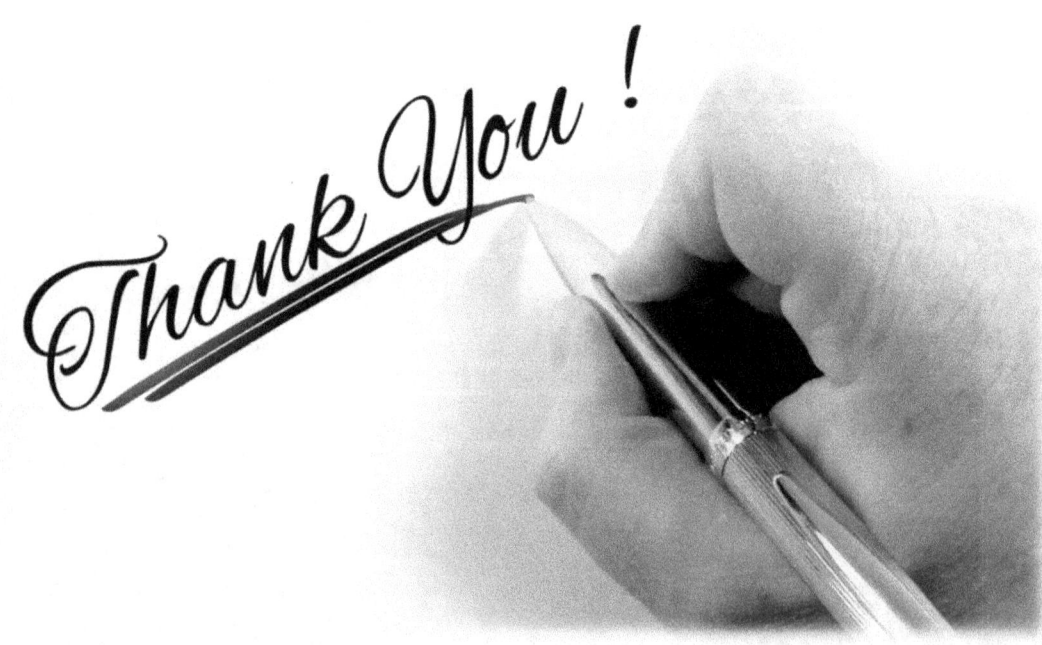